Foundations of YOGA

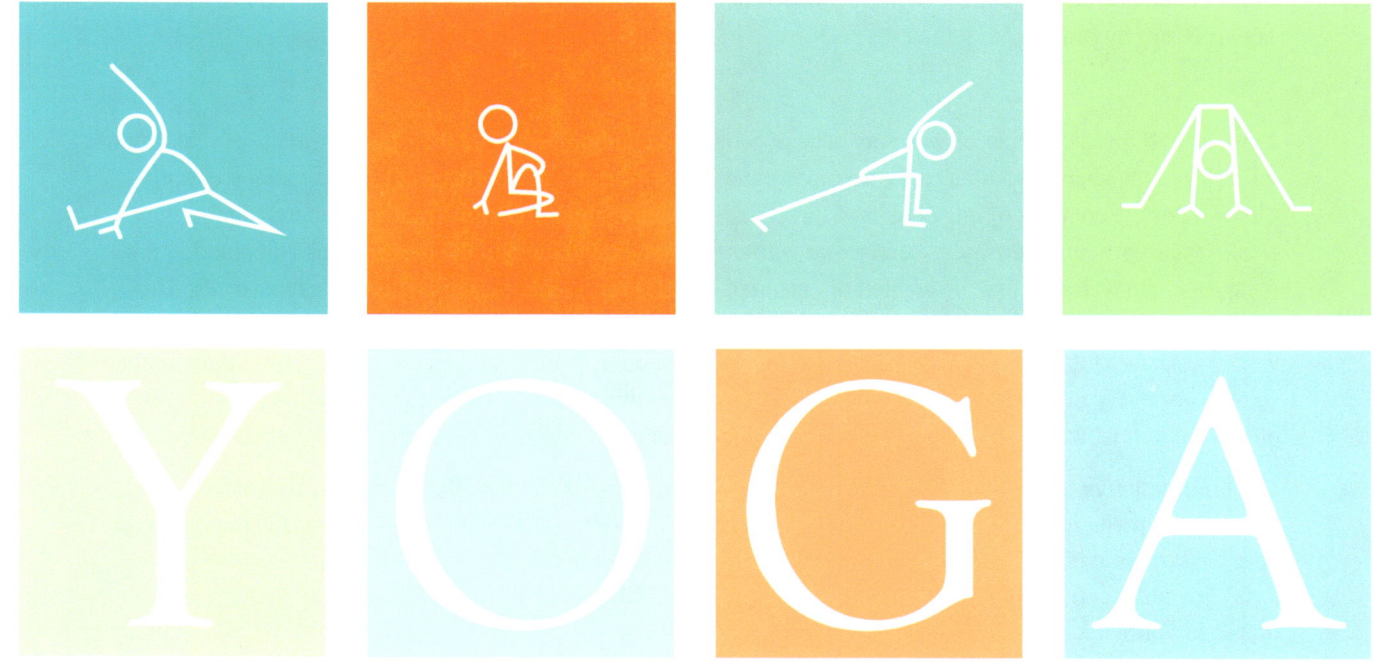

YOGA

Published by Trailhead Healing Arts Center, LLC

801 South Grand Avenue, West

Springfield, IL 62704 U.S.A.

www.trailheadcenter.org

Printed in the USA, 2014 by:

Capitol Blueprint

1313 S 1st St.

Springfield, IL 62704

The
Foundations
of
Yoga

Within creation are held in balance the three realms of body, mind, and spirit.

— Rig Veda

Introduction

This Foundations of Yoga booklet is designed to give you, a beginning Yoga student, some experience with the skills of Ashtanga, the eight limbs of Yoga. This is not an effort of your intellectual mind in learning these concepts; instead, set aside the intellectual process of learning and allow this learning to unfold naturally on a journey of self-discovery.

By now, you know that Yoga is not just an exercise program for the body, but a journey of the body, mind and spirit. It is a system to help you give up the habits of the body/mind and see what has always been there, if you just had a way to look. We hope that you use this booklet to enhance your Yoga practice.

Namaste,
Justina and all of the staff/teachers at Trailhead Healing Arts Center

Acknowledgements

Many students and faculty have knowingly and unknowingly assisted in developing this booklet. I would like to especially thank Mary Addison-Lamb for writing and publishing the first editions of this booklet, Miriam Pierson for many of the drawings and Stephen Newell for drafting the sections "Being a Good Yoga Student" and "Developing a Home Practice." Hernando Albarracin, Nancy Long and Nancy Ryan have taken the time to read, reflect, and suggest changes to the first drafts of the book. All of the students at Namaste/Trailhead Healing Arts have helped to form the words that convey the essence of Yoga in this booklet. Thanks to you all.

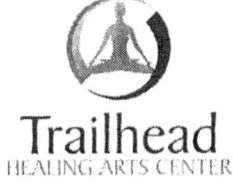

Trailhead
HEALING ARTS CENTER

The 8 Limbs (Ashtanga) of Yoga

The "skills" or "practices of yoga" you have experienced are:

1. Pratyahara—sense withdrawal
   The ability to relax and become intimately aware of the feelings and sensations of the body through guided body scans. This is the first part of practice. Moving your senses from the outside world to the inside world.

2. Pranayama—breath awareness
   The practice of 3-part breath. This breath cleanses the physical body, calms the emotional body and clears your mind so that you can make choices without the clouded judgment and critical habits you have developed.

3. Asana—postures
   Once you are deeply aware of the feelings of the body/mind, you can begin to move in, hold, and come out of the postures with awareness, noticing habits of movement and holding and experiencing the poses, just as you are, with a clearer sense of what you are able to explore safely and confidently.

4. Dharana—concentration
   Class gives you the opportunity to begin the practice of concentration, to see how the mind wanders away and upon, seeing that, bring it back to the object of attention over and over again.

5. Dhyana—meditation
   In the final relaxation, you have the opportunity to let go of the physical, emotional and intellectual self and open to the practice of allowing the mind to be "present," not in the past or in the future but in the present moment.

6. Samadhi
   In that present moment there is nothing but you and the Divine.

The two remaining limbs are Yama and Niyama, guidelines of how to treat others as well as yourself. We offer this exploration in the Foundation II and III.

Being a Good Yoga Student:
Some tips and etiquette when attending a Yoga class

- Practice barefoot, remove shoes.

- Wear comfortable and modest clothing. Avoid wearing excessive or jingly jewelry. Avoid perfume or cologne.

- Don't have a heavy meal within three hours; don't have a light meal within an hour of class.

- Go to the restroom before class.

- Leave cell phones outside the classroom and turned off.

- Arrive early. While waiting for class to start, keep classroom conversation to a minimum.

- Inform the teacher before class of any physical injuries or problems.

- If you arrive late (never more than 10 minutes), settle in as quietly as possible. Wait until the class is moving before unrolling a sticky mat. If you arrive in a rush, spend a few minutes quietly centering yourself before joining the class; let your frenzied mind catch up with your body.

- Sit close to the teacher if you have hearing difficulties.

- Pay attention to the teacher and follow the instructions given. If you do not understand something or you have a question, ask.

- Intend to have a beginner's mind—a mind that is open, an attitude of possibility, and the ability to see things as fresh and new. Yoga is self-exploration and self-discovery—not an exercise in power and control.

- Careful not to force or struggle. Honor your body/mind. If you need to rest during class, move into a quiet pose, such as child's pose or relaxation pose, until you are ready to re-join the class.

- Careful not to be competitive. This is an individual journey and comparing yourself to others misses the point.

- Stay for the entire class. Leaving early, especially before, or during, relaxation can be disruptive to nearby students. It also robs you of one of the best parts of class!

- Put away props neatly at the end of class.

- Sign up early for classes.

- During the last pose of class, shavasana, people turn so their feet are facing away from the teacher and their head toward him/her. In many studios around the world, this is done to show respect for the teacher.

Developing a Home Practice

Practice is basically the correct effort required to move toward, reach and maintain the state of Yoga. It is only when correct practice is followed for a long time, without interruptions and with a quality of positive attitude and eagerness, that it can succeed.

Yoga Sutra 1.13 and 1.14

Yoga is a commitment to be present to your physical, mental, and spiritual life. Changes occur slowly and your regular practice gives you experience staying open to those changes. Keep a balanced attitude and allow your practice to develop step-by-step.

Yoga is not about tying yourself into knots. Rather, it is about loosening all of your bodily, emotional and intellectual knots. Gradually and naturally, you will find yourself awakening to the higher values of life.

Intention

As you begin a home practice, set your goals. Decide why you want to practice Yoga. Base these goals on your needs. For example, you might want to work on certain postures, get rid of specific stiffness, strengthen a weakness, counter the effects of another activity such as working at a desk all day, improving your emotional well-being, or deepening your spirituality.

Keep these goals in mind, for they become the encouragement for your practice. When you feel like quitting or postponing your practice, remember your intentions.

Discipline

Developing a home practice requires courage, daring, perseverance, knowledge and faith. It is essential to practice daily until it becomes a habit. This may seem like an added burden or chore—something else to add to your already busy life. However, the benefits you receive will quickly change this from a chore to a natural and life-enhancing habit.

Stay for the long haul. There is no quick fix; it takes time and constant effort. The longer you practice Yoga, the more enjoyable and beneficial it becomes. It takes six weeks to make something a habit. You

should give your practice as least six months before you evaluate its effect.

Avoid making your practice a chore. Always do your best and do not worry about the outcome. Be diligent, but relaxed, in your approach.

Expect growth and change. Allow your Yoga practice to transform not only your body, but also your mind and your spirit. Gently work with your limitations and expand your abilities. Outgrow useless attitudes and negative thoughts. Discover new horizons.

Commitment

Make a commitment to your practice. Decide how often you will practice and how long each session will last. Keep your commitment simple and manageable. Be realistic and do not put yourself at a disadvantage by over-committing yourself and facing the struggle to meet any difficult goals.

Take a careful look at your strengths, limitations, and your environment. Consider your physical condition and other commitments in your life as you design a practice that meets your needs. Grow and deepen that practice over time, as you are ready.

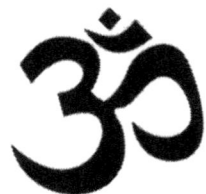

When to Practice

Choose a time of day that is best for your schedule and lifestyle. Usually, the best time to practice is either early in the morning, late afternoon, or before bed. It's best to practice at the same time every day.

Factors to consider when choosing a time:

- When are you least likely to be disturbed?
- When is it easiest for you to make time?
- Are you a morning person or evening person?
- Wait at least two hours after a meal.
- Morning as a way to greet and prepare for the day.
- Evening as a way to unwind.
- Understand you will be less flexible in the morning.
- An evening practice may energize you and make it more difficult to fall asleep.

In setting a schedule, be kind to yourself and be realistic. A daily practice is ideal. It is better to do a small amount of practice every day than it is to do a lot some days and nothing on other days.

Where to Practice

Find a quiet, peaceful, well-ventilated space where you will not be disturbed. Avoid drafty or cold rooms. The amount of the space needed isn't very large. As long as you can lie on the ground, reach your arms overhead and stretch your arms out to your side (T-position), that space is big enough.

Turn off the ringer on the phone and hang a "Do Not Disturb" sign on the door.

To improve your space:

- Bring a few favorite objects into the space: photographs, stones, flowers, and anything that reminds you of your spirit.
- Keep the space clean and uncluttered. Our external space mirrors our internal experience. Create an aesthetically pleasing space that will be a joy for you to practice in.
- Listen to inspiring music or open the windows to the sounds of life.
- Explore different smells in your space. Try candles, incense, and oils.
- Eliminate harsh, direct, and overhead lighting. Replace it with soft, indirect lighting.

How Long to Practice

At the start, thirty to sixty minutes is an ideal length of time for each practice. If you are pressed for time, try to take at least twenty minutes for a practice. On the weekends, or days when you have extra time, take longer—maybe an hour or more. It is better to have a consistent twenty minutes every day than to sporadically practice thirty to sixty minutes.

Every time you practice, set the length of time before you start and do at least that amount of time. Resist the temptation to quit early to work on some other task. Set your intention to practice and focus completely on it.

What to Practice

Allow your practice to grow and change based on your experiences. Challenge, or comfort, yourself as necessary. The asanas (postures) are tools to rejuvenate your body, to quiet your mind and to reveal your spirit. Practice the postures you feel are needed at this moment and make the modifications you feel are necessary.

As you practice, trust your intuition and instinct. If something does not feel right, do not continue. If your body says one thing and your mind says another, go with your body.

Your practice should adhere to the following order:

- Warm up, bring your awareness to your body and breath with centering and warm-up poses. Gently waken the spine and the body.
- Heating poses—standing or back-bending poses.
- Cooling poses—forward-bending or twisting poses.
- Pranayama/relaxation/meditation

Always incorporate a final relaxation and a meditation. This is the most important part of your practice. You should plan to spend at least five minutes in final relaxation for every thirty minutes of asanas. Your body/mind uses this time to integrate what was learned and find a new balance. Then, gradually come to a seated position for meditation, making sure that the head, neck and trunk of the body are in alignment. Focus on your breath, or personal mantra, for as long as you have time. Meditation guides your body/mind back to the Self and allows you to purify your consciousness.

How to Practice

You may find a standard routine very helpful to learn the poses and to notice your responses over time. Then, you might vary your routine as you look at the new habits you have developed. Approach each practice with the same intensity and freshness as your first session.

Focus on and enhance your awareness. Listen to your body. Move slowly but surely; never use jerky or fast movements. Practice at a slow, steady pace while calmly focusing on your breath and postural movements. Practice each pose to your own limits, savor the pose and be present. If you start to rush, ask yourself, "Why?"

In each pose, observe:

- What are my feelings?
- What are my sensations?
- What are my thoughts?
- What does the pose teach me about myself?
- What are the nuances of the breath?
- What are the details of the pose: position of feet, arms, head, spine, etc.?

Equipment

You can practice Yoga at home with no special equipment. The minimum you need is comfortable clothing.

A mat, strap, blanket and, if you wish, an eye pillow could be used. A non-slip mat helps give you stability in standing poses and some cushion for floor poses. A strap may help in some of the poses. A blanket serves two purposes: folded, you can use it to elevate your seat for some of the forward-bending and twisting poses and, unfolded, to cover yourself during relaxation. If you are on a tight budget, a large towel or rug can be used as a mat, an old necktie can be used as a strap, and a sock filled with rice can be used as an eye pillow.

Ritual

Your habit and your intention will be improved if you involve some ritual with your practice. The daily ritual of unfolding your mat signals your body to prepare for and focus on your practice. Likewise, lighting a candle or incense, can send a signal to your mind and spirit that it is time to focus on your practice.

Excuses

Try not to let your practice be disrupted by your daily life. Nor should houseguests, vacations, travel, kids home for the summer, mild illness and other changes in your daily pattern interrupt your practice. Some thoughts on these:

- If you have guests in your home, or your home is too crowded, try going outside and find a secluded place to practice, getting up thirty minutes earlier than everyone else, or go to another building to practice, such as an empty room in your office building.

- When traveling, Yoga is an easy fitness routine to maintain. You can do your practice in your hotel room. Stranded with a long layover at an airport? Find a deserted gate area and do some asanas.

- When you are visiting another city, find a Yoga class. Drop in. You will meet some nice people and learn new techniques.

- Illness does not need to stop your practice. You may be able to practice breathing and relaxation. With a cold or other minor ailment, you can do a number of very gentle poses.

- Practice with a partner or a group of friends. Encourage each other.

- Do not let apathy or procrastination stop your practice. If you have a day where you just do not feel like it, practice anyway! Coping with moments like these is part of your growing process and will give you an opportunity to observe and learn about yourself.

Most importantly, enjoy your practice! Make it pleasurable and fun!

A Breath for Relaxation

The "Yoga" Breath
3-part breath/diaphragmatic breathing

The most important "tool" in the yoga toolbox is the breath. The breath is your link between the conscious mind and the unconscious mind. When you return the unconscious breathing process to your consciousness, your consciousness expands to include the feelings and sensations of the body/mind. When you become aware of the feelings and sensations, you can begin to be conscious of the habits of the body/mind. And when you bring your habits into your awareness, you can begin to make choices out of your conscious mind instead of the unconscious mind.

If you are attentive to your actions, you are not a prisoner of your habits.

In the Foundation Series, you begin to notice the breath and to practice feeling the 3-part breath. Not only does this use the entire capacity of the breath, but also it is a signal to the body/mind to relax. You can feel the body/mind relax in just 3 breaths! Always breathe in and out of the nostrils.

The primary muscle of breathing is the diaphragm, as illustrated below. When you breath in, it moves down to draw the breath in. When you breathe out, the diaphragm moves up to push the breath out.

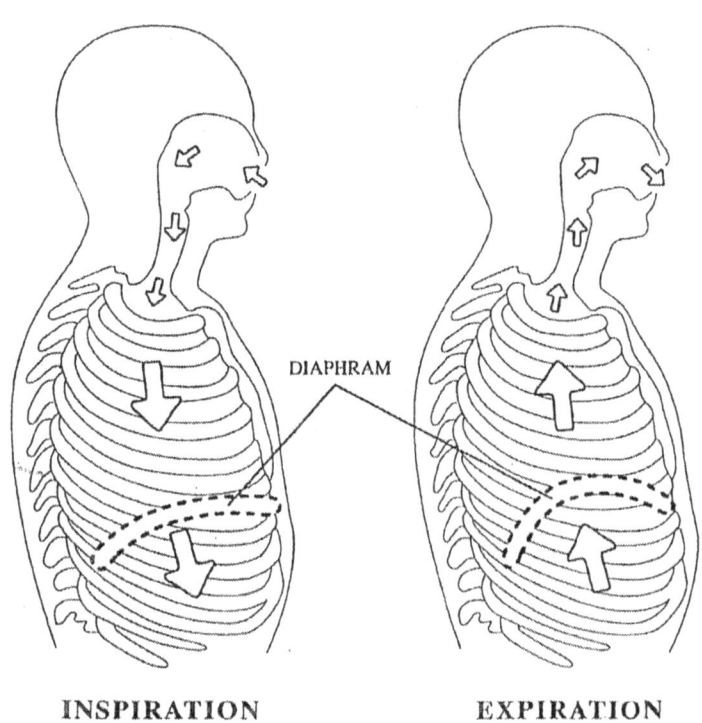

DIAPHRAM

INSPIRATION   EXPIRATION

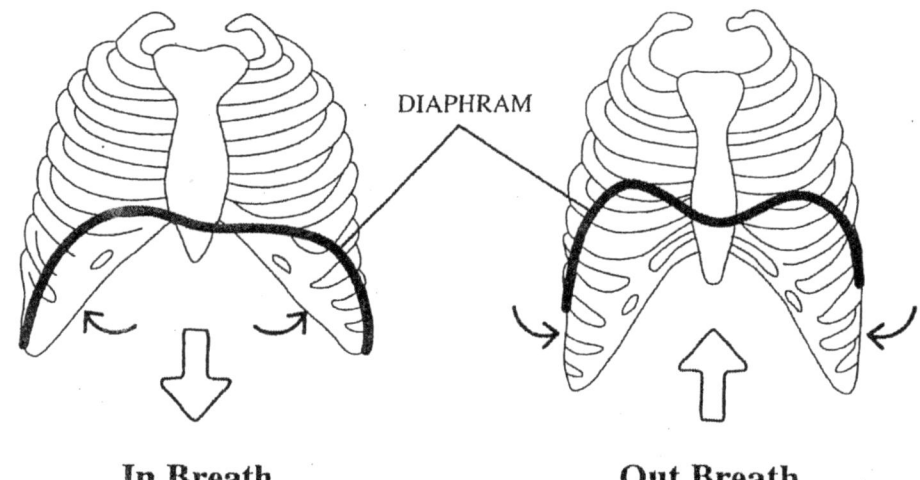

In Breath   **Out Breath**

To make this breath a habit, take your hands to your belly (below the navel) and feel the belly expand as you breathe in and condense as you breathe out. When this feels natural, move your hands to embrace your low ribs and feel the breath fill your belly and then expand your ribs. When this feels natural, move your hands to the top of the chest with your fingers just below the collarbone and experience the breath filling to the top of the chest and the breastbone rising.

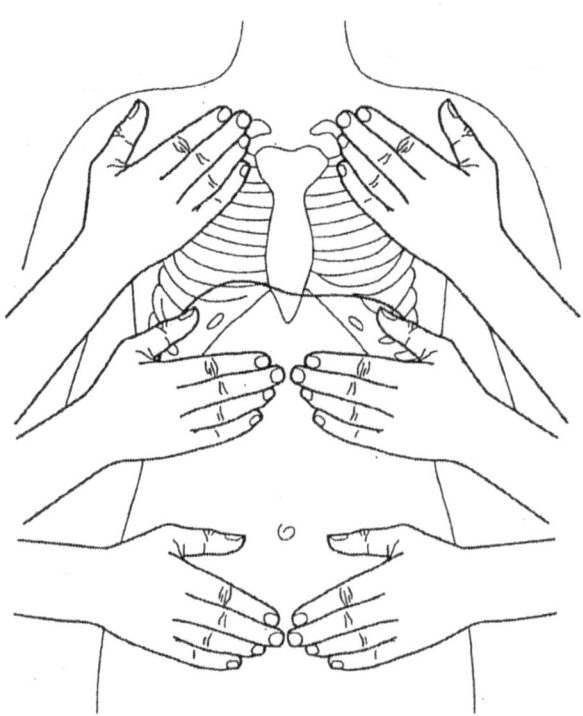

3-Part Breath

When this becomes a habit, you will find that your breath is your first action to bring yourself home. Home is where your mind, body and spirit are truly *present*, not in the future or in the past but in the present moment. When you are in this place, you will be at your best…confident, competent and at peace.

Namaste….when you are in that place in you, and I am in that place in me, we are one.

Practice Outlines

Foundation Practices

These are outlines for six days of practice. Completing them assures you that all the body/mind has had its "turn" for the week.

Day 1

I. *Centering: Body/Breath Awareness (Hold for as long as you wish.)*
Relaxation Pose with 3-part breath
Easy Seated Pose
Neck Stretches/Flower Open
Mountain Pose
Crescent Moon Series: *(Hold each pose for at least 3 breaths.)*
- Side-to-Side Arch
- Supported Back Arch
- Supported Forward Bend

II. *Heating Asanas (Hold for at least 3 breaths.)*
Tree
Warrior I
Child's Pose: Extended
Airplane

III. *Cooling Asanas (Hold for as long as you wish.)*
Pelvic Rock
Knee to Chest
Knee Down Twist
Hamstring Stretch with Tie

IV. *Relaxation*

Day 2

I. *Centering: Body/Breath Awareness (Hold for as long as you wish.)*
Relaxation Pose with 3-part breath
Easy Seated Pose
Neck Stretches/Flower Open
Mountain Pose
Crescent Moon Series:
- Side-to-Side Arch
- Supported Back Arch
- Supported Forward Bend

II. *Heating Asanas (Hold for at least 3 breaths.)*
Tree
Warrior II
Triangle
Child's Pose: Extended
Cobra I

III. *Cooling Asanas (Hold for as long as you wish.)*
Pelvic Rock
Knee to Chest
Knee Down Twist
Hamstring Stretch with Tie

IV. *Relaxation*

Day 3

I. *Centering: Body/Breath Awareness (Hold for as long as you wish.)*
Relaxation Pose with 3-part breath
Easy Seated Pose
Neck Stretches/Flower Open
Mountain Pose
Crescent Moon Series:
- Side-to-Side Arch
- Supported Back Arch
- Supported Forward Bend

II. *Heating Asanas (Hold for at least 3 breaths.)*
Tree
Warrior I
Warrior II
Child's Pose: Extended
Airplane

III. *Cooling Asanas (Hold for as long as you wish.)*
Pelvic Rock
Knee to Chest
Knee Down Twist
Hamstring Stretch with Tie

IV. *Relaxation*

Day 4

I. *Centering: Body/Breath Awareness (Hold for as long as you like.)*
Seated Pose with 3-part breath
Eye exercises
Six Movements of the Spine
   • Cat Stretch
   • Thread-the-Needle
   • Wag the Tail

II. *Heating Asanas (Hold for at least 3 breaths.)*
½ Sunbird
Stork
Chair
Sun Salutation
   • Shoulders Rolled Back & Down
   • Downward/Upward Roll
   • Lunge
   • Downward Facing Dog
   • Cobra I

III. *Cooling Asanas (Hold for as long as you wish.)*
Butterfly/Cobbler's Pose (seated)
Supported Seated Forward Fold
Tranquility Pose/Legs-up-the-wall

IV. *Relaxation*

Day 5

I. *Centering: Body/Breath Awareness (Hold for as long as you like.)*
Seated Pose with 3-part breath
Eye exercises
Six Movements of the Spine
   • Cat Stretch
   • Thread-the-Needle
   • Wag the Tail

II. *Heating Asanas (Hold for at least 3 breaths.)*
½ Sunbird
Stork
Chair
Sun Salutation
   • Shoulders Rolled Back & Down
   • Downward/Upward Roll
   • Lunge
   • Downward Facing Dog
   • Cobra I
Supported Fish

III. *Cooling Asanas (Hold for as long as you wish.)*
Seated Twist
Tranquility Pose/Legs-up-the-wall

IV. *Relaxation*

Day 6

I. *Centering: Body/Breath Awareness (Hold for as long as you like.)*
Seated Pose with 3-part breath
Eye exercises
Six Movements of the Spine
   • Cat Stretch
   • Thread-the-Needle
   • Wag the Tail

II. *Heating Asanas (Hold for at least 3 breaths.)*
Stork
Chair
Sun Salutation
   • Shoulders Rolled Back & Down
   • Downward/Upward Roll
   • Lunge
   • Downward Facing Dog
   • Cobra I
Supported Fish

III. *Cooling Asanas (Hold for as long as you wish.)*
Butterfly/Cobbler's Pose (seated)
Seated Twist
Supported Seated Forward Fold

IV. *Relaxation*

Easy Seated Pose (Sukhasana)

- This is the starting pose from which all other seated poses evolve.
- Make a firm foundation sitting on a zafu, folded blanked or other firm cushion.
- Allow the knees to fold the heels in without resting the legs on one another.
- Rest the weight on the sitz bones with the knees dropping below the hipbones.
- Tailbone should be pointed down and not under.
- Let the spine curve up, shoulders dropping down and back, letting the heart center open.
- Extend the back of the neck, allowing the chin to become parallel with the earth.
- Breathe up and down the spine until you feel at rest in the pose.

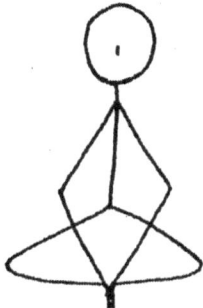

Fig. 1: Easy Seated Pose (Sukhasana)

Neck/Shoulder Stretches

- Begin in an Easy-Seated Pose (Fig. 1). Allow the head to drop forward, chin to the chest, resist allowing the shoulders to roll forward. Just allow the weight of the head to open the back of the neck and shoulders.
- Breathe into the stretch...with each in-breath, sense and feel and with each out-breath, let go a little more. Count at least 8 breaths.
- Roll the head to the right, bringing the right ear over the shoulder, left ear toward the ceiling, then turn the head to look down toward the right knee.
- Breathe into the stretch...with each in-breath, sense and feel and with each out-breath, let go a little more. Count at least 8 breaths.
- Let the head roll back forward and up to the left bringing the left ear over the shoulder, right ear toward the ceiling, then turn the head to look down toward the left knee.
- Breathe into the stretch...with each in-breath, sense and feel and with each out-breath, let go a little more. Count at least 8 breaths.
- Let the head roll back forward. Repeat as necessary.
- Bring the head back up to be supported over the shoulders and feel the opening in the neck and shoulders.

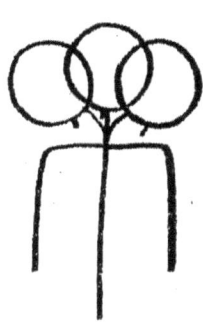

Fig. 2: Neck/Shoulder Stretches

Shoulder Rolls

- Begin in Easy Seated Pose (Fig. 1).
- Bring the attention to the right shoulder.
- As you breathe in, allow the shoulder to roll forward and up and on the exhale let the shoulder roll back and down.
- Continue to roll the shoulder feeling the shoulder opening and relaxing. Make big smooth movements. Use the breath to move you.
- Allow the whole arm to move. Allow the head and neck to move in whatever way feels comfortable.
- Reverse the direction. Breathing in, roll the shoulder back and up, exhaling bring it forward and down.
- Repeat other side.

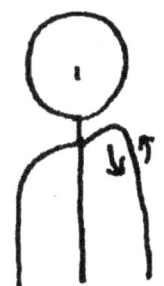

Fig. 3: Shoulder Rolls

Flower Opening (Shoulders, Chest and Back)

- Begin in Easy Seated Pose (Fig. 1).
- Let the head come forward, chin to the chest. Interlace the fingers and place the hands at the back of the neck.
- With an in-breath, slowly lift the head, letting the elbows stretch back and open, sliding the hands up to the back of the head.
- Lay the head in the hands, with the back of the neck lengthened.
- Drop the shoulders down and back, and feel the shoulder blades moving down and in and the front of the chest stretching open.
- Exhale and fold back forward to the opening position.

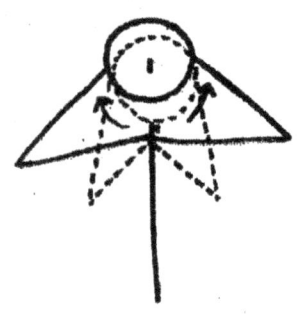

Fig. 4: Flower Opening
(Shoulders, Chest and Back)

Yoga Mudra

- Come to your knees and sit back to your heels.
- Reach the arms around back and interlace the fingers.
- Keep the elbows bent and push the hands back to squeeze the shoulder blades together.
- Drop the shoulders down and back and lower the chin into the chest.
- Hold for several long, easy breaths.

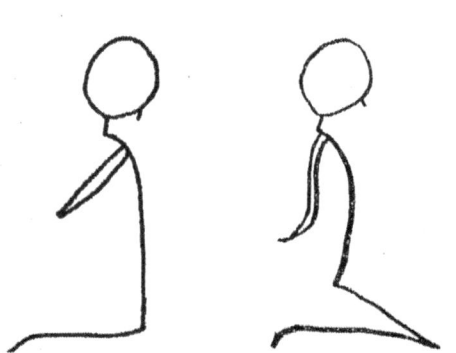

Fig. 5: Yoga Mudra

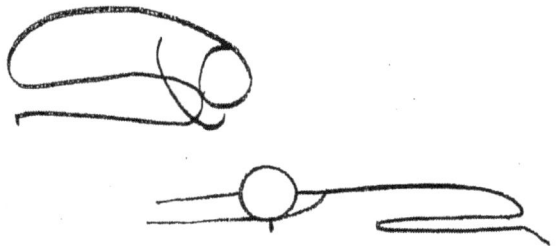

Fig. 6: Child's Pose (Balasana)

Child's Pose (Balasana)

- Come on to your knees and sit the hips back to the heels.
- Allow the knees to be apart while the big toes are together.
- Fold the torso forward to rest on the thighs and bring the head to rest on folded forearms, or rest your head on the floor and lay your arms alongside your legs.
- Encourage the breath to be long and deep.

Extended Child's Pose (Balasana)

- As above with the arms actively stretched out on the floor in front.

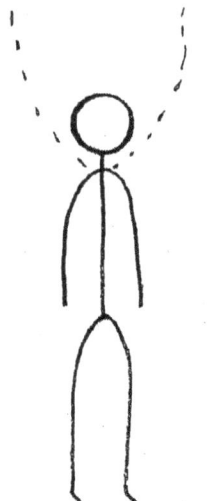

Fig. 7: Mountain Pose (Tadasana)

Mountain Pose (Tadasana)

- This is the basic standing pose from which all the standing poses evolve.
- Stand with feet parallel and pressing into the earth. Body drawing upward, knees soft, kneecaps lifting, thighs hugging toward the bones as the pelvic floor lifts, the tail bone slightly tucks under the torso.
- Torso lifting up out of the hips, lifting at the breastbone, lifting at the back of the head.
- Spine lengthening, crown of the head lifting.
- Arms long and straight. Shoulders relaxed down and back.
- Breathe along the body, feeling the simultaneous movement of energy down into the earth and up into the sky.
- Feel the body aligning, resisting gravity perfectly…as if you could stand here forever.
- Feel yourself gradually becoming aligned ear over the shoulder, over the hip, over the knee, over the ankle. Weight resting just in front of the ankle and dropping to the center of the heel.

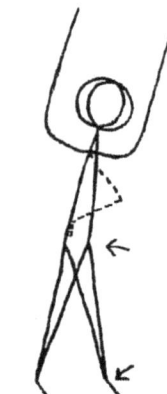

Fig. 8: Crescent Moon Series (Ardha Chandrasana):
Supported Lateral Bend

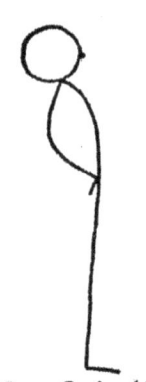

Fig. 9: Crescent Moon Series (Ardha Chandrasana):
Supported Upper Back Arch

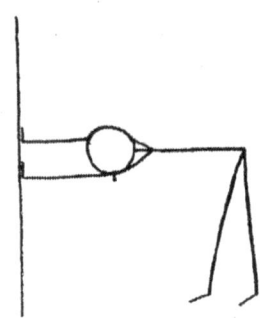

Fig. 10: Crescent Moon Series (Ardha Chandrasana):
Supported Forward Fold at the Wall

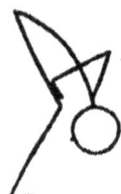

Fig. 11: Crescent Moon Series (Ardha Chandrasana):
Supported Forward Fold on the Thighs

Crescent Moon Series: (Ardha Chandrasana)

1. **Supported Lateral Bend**
   - Standing in Mountain Pose (Fig. 7). place the left hand on the hip.
   - Take a breath in as you stretch the right arm up and allow the shoulder to rest down. Shift the weight to the right leg and let the right hip drift out.
   - Stretch up and long as you arch to the left. Keep the body in one plane. Focus on the lengthening of the body and allow the arc to be a natural extension of that length.
   - Press the feet into the earth.
   - Return to Tadasana. Repeat other side.

2. **Supported Upper Back Arch**
   - Begin in Tadasana (Mountain Pose) (Fig. 7)
   - Take the hands to support the low back by placing palms on the waist. Squeeze knees up, tuck tail under, stabilizing the lower part of the body from the waist down.
   - Take a breath in and, as you exhale, stretch up and back, bringing the breath to the front of the spine. Lift at the navel, lift at the breast-bone. Keep the chin toward the chest.
   - Take the breath into the spine and allow it to gently release.
   - Return to Tadasana.

3a. **Supported Forward Fold (at the Wall)**
   - Place the hands on the wall about waist high.
   - Walk backward while bending forward until your torso is parallel to the floor.
   - Bend the knees and take the tailbone back and up.
   - Take the crown of the head forward and the ears next to the arms.
   - Soften the shoulders away from the ears and breathe.
   - To come up, take a breath and step one foot forward.

3b. **Supported Forward Fold (on the Thighs) (Uttanasana)**
   - Allow the head to roll forward and release the spine forward one vertebra at a time.
   - Roll the pelvis forward, pointing the tailbone toward the sky. Rest the belly on the thighs and let the head dangle forward.
   - To come up, uncurl the spine one vertebra at a time. Let the head come up last.

Pelvic Rock

- Lie on the floor with your feet drawn up just behind the buttocks. Arms resting alongside the body.
- Draw a breath in and allow the low back to lift off the floor while the tailbone drops down…creating a little tunnel under the upper back and the hips.
- With the out breath, rock the low back down and press the waist into the floor and feel the tailbone tilt up.
- Continue rocking the pelvis, allowing the breath to lead the movement.
- Feel the belly tighten when the waist presses down.
- Feel the back tighten when the waist lifts up.

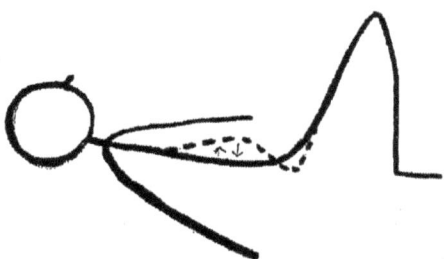

Fig. 12: Pelvic Rock

Knee Hug (Apanasana)

- Lie on the floor, bring both feet up behind the buttocks (alt. leave the left leg stretched out along the floor), draw the right knee up and into the chest and embrace it with your arms.
- Allow the breath to deepen so that the belly massages into the thigh and the thigh into the belly.
- Repeat other side.

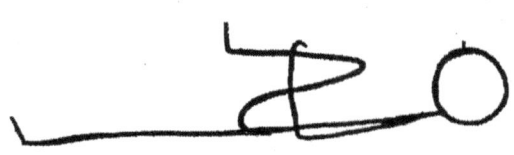

Fig. 13: Knee Hug (Apanasana)

Knee-down Twist (var. Jathara Parivartanasana)

- Lie down on the back and stretch the body long.
- Bring the arms into a "T" position.
- Bring the sole of right foot onto the left knee.
- Take a breath in and, as you exhale, roll the right knee towards the floor on your left side.
- Place your left hand on right knee and allow the weight of your arm to deepen the twist.
- Keep right arm out in "T" position.
- Keep both shoulders on the floor.
- Turn to look at your right hand. Relax and breathe for several breaths.
- Repeat other side.

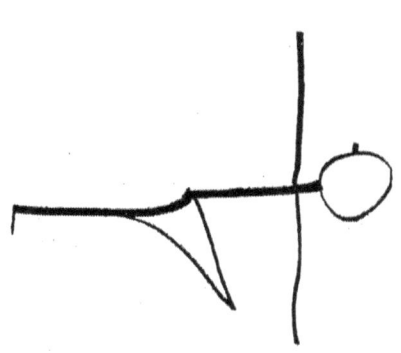

Fig. 14: Knee-down Twist (var. Jathara Parivartanasana)

Face the long edge of the mat.

Hamstring Stretch with a Tie

- The very best way to stretch out the hamstrings, *if done properly.*
- Lie on your back with both knees drawn up behind the buttocks, feet on the floor.
- Place a strap around the heel or ball, of the right foot.
- Extend the leg fully along the floor pressing the heel away and point the toes toward the nose.
- Slowly and carefully raise the foot toward the ceiling.
- Keep the leg straight until you find the stretch in the hip and leg.
- Hold and breathe to the stretch for at least 15 breaths.
- Repeat other side.

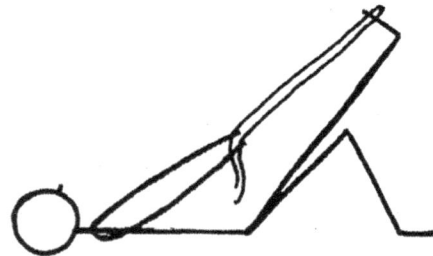

Fig. 15: Hamstring Stretch with a Tie

Crocodile (Makarasana)

- Come to rest on the belly with the toes turned out/or in.
- Prop the shoulders up on the elbows.
- Fold the arms, fingertips to opposite elbow, and resting on the forearms.
- Slide the arms forward just until you can rest the forehead on the forearms.
- Feel the breath in the belly, ribs and all the way to the shoulders. Feel the breath in the back body, filling the low, mid and upper back.

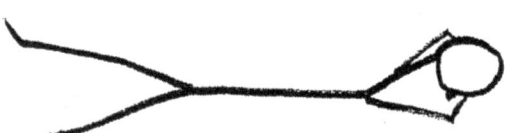

Fig. 16: Crocodile (Makarasana)

½ Sunbird (Chakravakasana)

- Begin in table position. Take a breath and, as you exhale, bring the right knee towards the chest while you drop the head down to bring nose toward the knee.
- On the in-breath, extend the right heel back as you extend the leg, extending the crown of the head forward. Drop the shoulders away from the ears.
- Breathe and hold.
- Repeat other side.

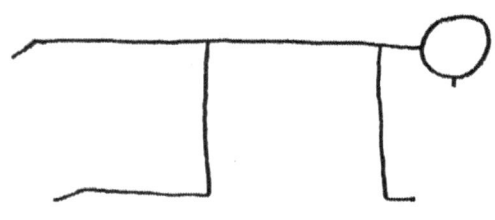

Fig. 17: ½ Sunbird (Chakravakasana)

Warrior II (Virabhadrasana)

- Face the long edge of the mat.
- Separate the legs one full leg length apart. Hips facing forward.
- Turn the right heel in, the left heel out.
- Bring the right knee directly over the ankle, and keep the torso perpendicular.
- Engage the legs by pressing both feet into the earth and draw the back knee up into the thigh.
- Raise the right arm to shoulder height and lengthen, left hand on hip or stretched on the same line behind.
- Draw the rear shoulder/arm slightly back and turn the head to gaze over the forward hand.
- Extend both legs equally away from the center of gravity and allow that center to gently rest towards the Earth.
- Repeat other side.

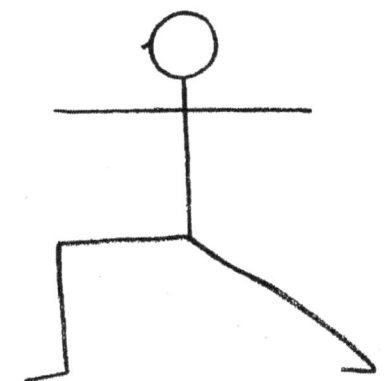

Fig. 18: Warrior II (Virabhadrasana)

Airplane (var. Adho Mukha Navasana)

- Come to rest on the belly, arms in "T" position, legs stretched out behind.
- With an in-breath, extend the legs back and lift up, and lift the shoulders and the arms, palms down.
- Keep the head in a neutral position, back of the neck long, crown of the head reaching forward.
- Feel the back muscles tightening and lifting legs, arms and head.
- Reach back as much as you're lifting up.
- Hold and breathe for as long as it is comfortable.
- Release and let the breath wash through the back.

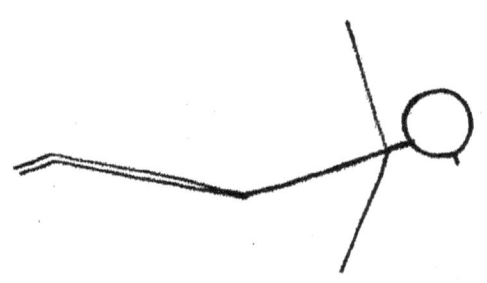

Fig. 19: Airplane (var. Adho Mukha Navasana)

Yoga Sit-up (full and ½)

- Interlace the fingers behind the head.
- Begin Pelvic Rock, and as you exhale, press the low back into the floor and lift the shoulders and the head.
- On the in breath, rest the head and arms back to the floor and lift the low back.
- Count the breaths. Take care not to pull on the head and neck but feel the belly muscles draw the pubic bone toward the nose. For the ½ sit ups, leave the left hand behind the head and take the right hand under the right knee and continue the sit-ups. Repeat other side.

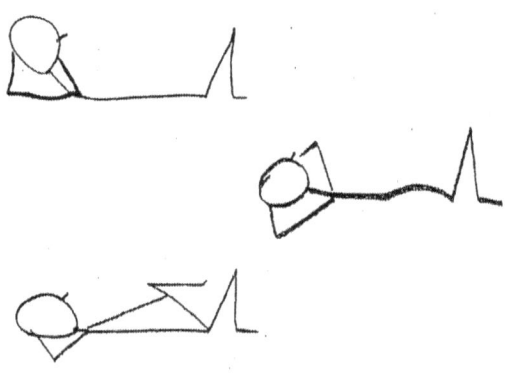

Fig. 20: Yoga Sit-up (full and ½)

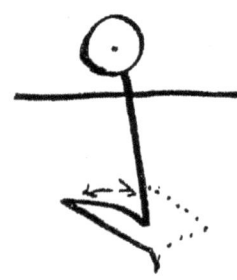

Fig. 21: Knee drops (var. Jathara Parivartanasana)

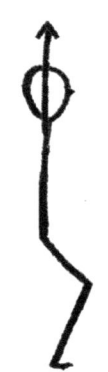

Fig. 22: Chair (Utkatasana)

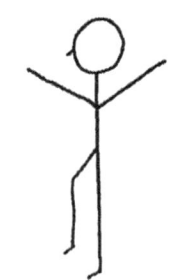

Fig. 23: Stork (var. Vrikshasana)

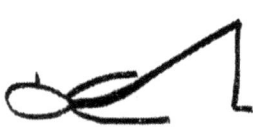

Fig. 24: Easy Bridge (Setu Bandha Sarvangasana)

Knee drops (var. Jathara Parivartanasana)

- Lay on your back, arms in "T" position.
- Bring the feet up just behind the buttocks.
- Take a breath and, as you exhale, let the knees roll to the right, roll your head to the left and turn the left palm up, right palm down.
- In breath, bring the knees and head up and roll the knees to the left, rolling the head to the right, turning the arms, and turning the hands.
- Continue for several breaths from side to side.
- Keep the feet on the floor until you feel strong enough to bring the knees up while keeping the low back pressing into the floor.

Powerful Pose (Utkatasana)

- Stand in Mountain Pose (Fig 7).
- Extend arms straight up and bring together without bending elbows.
- Exhale, bend the knees, lowering hips toward the floor.
- Avoid rounding the back.
- Hold for as many breaths as you are comfortable.

Stork (var. Vrikshasana)

- Begin in Mountain Pose (Fig. 7).
- Shift the weight over to the right side, press down and simultaneously lift up.
- Bring the left big toe to the floor next to the right foot.
- Raise the left knee up toward the chest and hold.
- Raise the arms and express yourself as a stork.
- Hold and breathe.
- Repeat other side.

Easy Bridge (Setu Bandha Sarvangasana)

- Begin with Pelvic Rock (Fig 12).
- When you feel the low back press into the floor and feel the tailbone tilt up, press the feet into the floor and allow the tailbone to gently lift the spine up off the floor, one vertebra at a time.
- Rest on the shoulders, draw the chin into the throat, and breathe long easy breaths for as long as it is comfortable.
- Roll back down, one vertebra at a time; tailbone is the last to touch the floor.

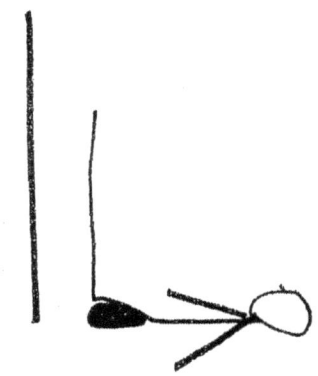

Fig. 25: Supported Tranquility
(var. Viparita Karani)

Fig. 26: Supine Crescent Moon

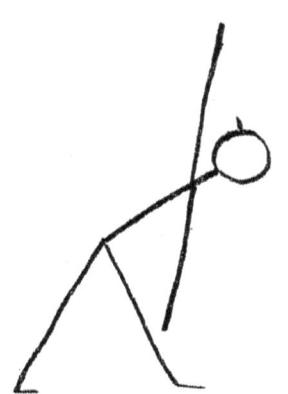

Fig. 27: Triangle (Trikonasana)

Supported Tranquility (var. Viparita Karani)

- Sit the left hip along side the wall.
- Come down onto the right forearm and swing the legs up the wall as you lower yourself onto your back.
- Push the feet into the wall and lift the hips up placing a *firm* bolster under the hips and low back.
- Bring the legs away from the wall and let them hang effortlessly.
- Bring the chin down toward the throat, lengthening the back of the neck.
- Close your eyes and take long and easy breaths for as long as you wish.

Supine Crescent Moon

- Stretch out on your back with your arms overhead.
- Walk the heels to the right and swing your arms to the right, leaving both the shoulders and hips on the floor.
- Hold and breathe to open the left side.
- Repeat other side.

Triangle (Trikonasana)

- Standing toward the long edge of the mat.
- Step the feet apart at least a full leg length apart hips facing forward. Press feet evenly into the earth, lengthen the legs, and pull up on the kneecaps.
- Turn the right heel in (90°), the left heel back and out (45°).
- Place the left hand on the hip. Stretch the right arm to the side over the right foot.
- Cock the left hip back and extend the right arm over the foot.
- Breathe in and as you exhale, stretch out over the right foot, lengthening the right rib cage, keeping the shoulders parallel to the wall behind you.
- Reach long through the right arm as you push the left hip up and back.
- Lower the right hand down to the leg.
- Bring the left arm vertically into the air.
- Turn the gaze toward the up-stretched hand. Hold and breathe.
- Repeat other side.

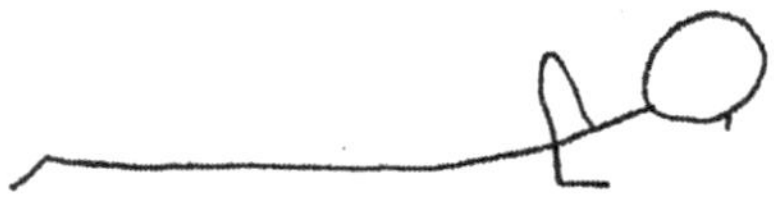

Cobra I (Bhujangasana)

- Lie on your belly, body long, and fingertips on the floor even with top edge of the shoulders. Big toes touching.
- Press the palms firmly into the earth, fingers are spread wide and firm with the index fingers pointing forward.
- Draw the belly button toward the sacrum and hold.
- With an in-breath, lift shoulders and head from the mid-back; naturally extending the spine forward and up.
- Keep the shoulders relaxed and allow the head and neck to remain neutral. Keep the shoulders away from the ears and the elbows hugged into the sides.
- Draw the torso forward and up, lengthening and lifting.
- Allow the head to be naturally lifted upward.
- Hold and breathe and make it easy.

Fig. 28: Cobra I

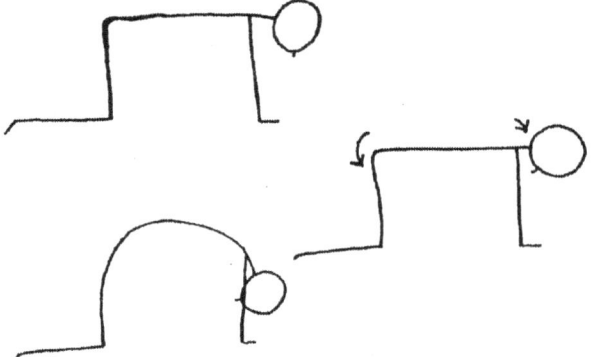

Fig. 29: Cat Stretches

1. **Cat Stretches**
   - Beginning in Table position, hands directly under the shoulders (or a little in front if the wrists are uncomfortable), knees directly under the hips, hip-width wide.
   - Take a breath and, on the exhale, drop tailbone and head toward the ground, lift the upper back toward the sky like a "Halloween cat."
   - In-breath back to table.

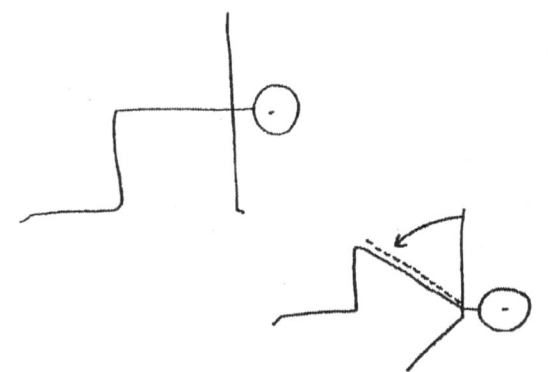

Fig. 30: Thread the Needle

2. **Thread the Needle**
   - Beginning in Table position, sweep the right arm up, extending from the heart center.
   - Bring the right arm down and tuck under the torso, threading between the left hand and the left knee, resting the right shoulder on the floor or a firm pillow. Assure yourself the neck and head are comfortable.
   - Extend the left arm toward the ceiling and roll the shoulder around.
   - Rest the hand over toward the right hip and breathe into this simple inverted twist.
   - Repeat other side.

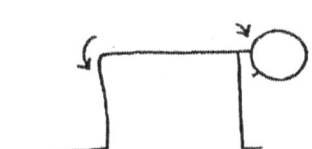

Fig. 31: Wag the Tail

3. **Wag the Tail**
   - Wag your tail to the right and look around your right shoulder at your right hip.
   - Feel the squeeze in the right and the opening on the left side. Hold and breathe.
   - Repeat other side. (You can also stretch the left leg back and cross over right calf and press the top of the foot into the floor to encourage the opening.)

Down Dog (Adho Mukha Svanasana)

- Beginning in Table position, curl the toes under and lift the hips up and back, lifting the tailbone up and lengthening through the arms.
- Beginners should keep the knees bent and focus on lengthening the line between the palms of the hands and the tailbone.
- Widen the upper back and relax the head face and neck, keeping the ears next to the arms.
- Lift the tailbone up. Tighten the belly.
- Hold and breathe. You might walk the feet down stretching out the back of the legs.

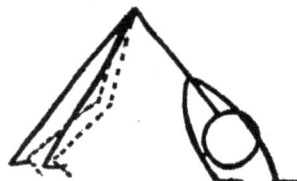

Fig. 32: Down Dog (Adho Mukha Svanasana)

Warrior I (Virabhadrasana)

- Step the right foot back to a 45° angle and squeeze the right knee up.
- Bring the pelvis into position by drawing the pubic bone up and engaging the belly.
- Take a breath, and as you exhale bring the left knee directly over the ankle.
- Take the arms forward and up and drop the shoulders down.
- Lift at the heart center, look forward, hold, and breathe.
- Repeat other side.

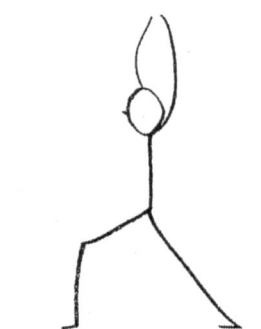

Fig. 33: Warrior I (Virabhadrasana)

Supported Fish (Matsyasana)

- Roll up a towel or a blanket.
- Place it under your back about level with your armpits, just below the tips of the shoulder blades.
- Lay back, supporting your head on the way down.
- Take your arms into "T" position.
- Soften into the pose and breathe.
- Hold for as long as you wish.

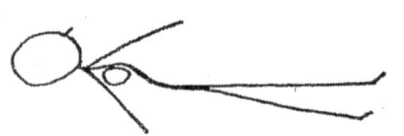

Fig. 34: Supported Fish (Matsyasana)

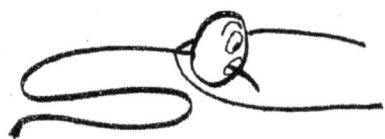

Fig. 35: Lion (Simhasana)

Lion (Simhasana)

- Sit back on your heels.
- Take a breath and, as you growl, stretch forward with your arms as you stick your tongue out and open your eyes real wide.
- Hold and breathe. Do a couple of times stretching the face, hands and shoulders.

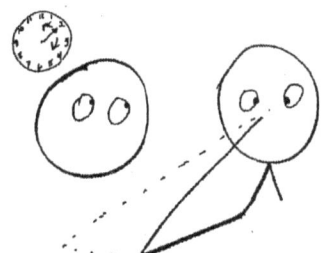

Fig. 36: Eye Exercises

Eye exercises

- Imagine a big clock face. Hold your head steady and allow your eyes to look up to 12. Feel the eyes stretching as you look all around the clock face, resting on each number. Move clockwise 4 times and then counterclockwise 4 times.
- Stretch your arm out and look at 2 fingers as you slowly bring them in to touch your nose and back out again.

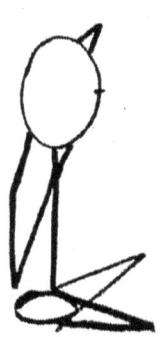

Fig. 37: Cow Face Pose (Gomukhasana)

Cow Face Pose (Gomukhasana)

- In Easy Seated Pose, take the left arm straight up over your head, bend the elbow and let your hand come to the center of your upper back.
- Bring the right arm along side the body and bend the elbow to let the left hand find the right. (Use a strap if your hands don't reach).
- Allow the shoulders to rest down and don't force or struggle but allow the breath to take your awareness into the stretch and allow the arms to come onto the same plane.
- Hold and breathe.
- Repeat other side.

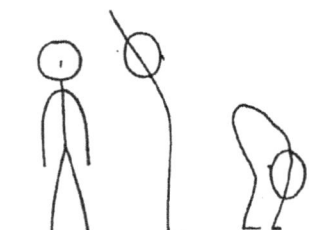

Fig. 38: Sun Salutation, steps 1-4

Sun Salutation (Surya Namaskar)

1. Begin in Mountain Pose (Fig. 7).
2. Swing the arms down and up to greet the "sun." In breath.
3. Allow the feet through the pelvis to be strong so that the upper chest can open up, shoulders dropping back and down in a standing back arch.
4. Exhale bend forward to come into a forward bend, resting on the thighs.

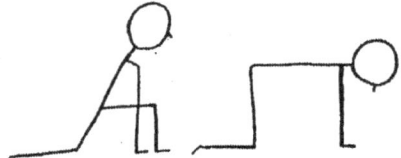

Fig. 39: Sun Salutation, step 5

5. With the hands next to the feet, step the left foot back and knee to the ground and come into a lunge position. Breathe. Check to make sure the right knee is directly over the ankle. Drop the weight into the hips and reach the heart center forward and up. Figure 39.

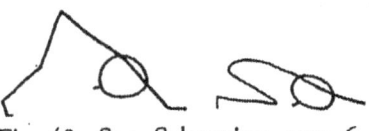

Fig. 40: Sun Salutation, step 6

6. Step back into table position. In-breath, lift the hips up and back into Down Dog posture.

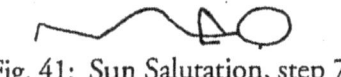

Fig. 41: Sun Salutation, step 7

7. Come down to the knees, sit back to your heels and slither forward onto your belly.

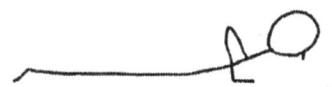

Fig. 42: Sun Salutation, step 8

8. Cobra I, fingertips even with the shoulders, pelvis locked, big toes together. In-breath, forward and up, using only the back muscles, lift torso; head and back neutral.

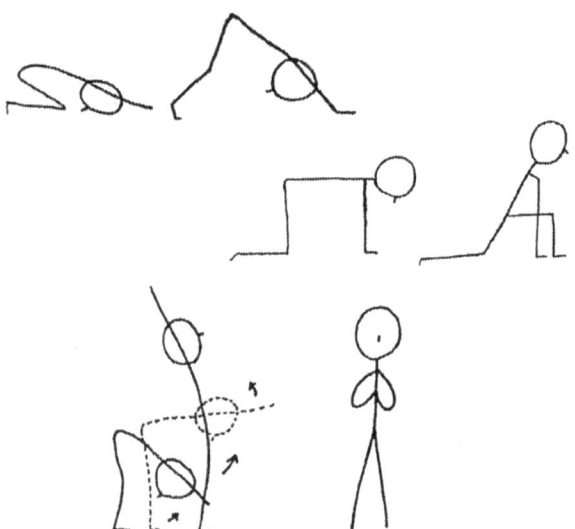

Fig. 43: Sun Salutation, step 9

9. Reverse...Push up into table, into downdog, back to table, step left foot forward into lunge, step right foot forward into forward bend, and with an in-breath, hinge at the hips to come up raising the arms in a big sweep and back to Mountain Pose.

10. Repeat other side.

Tree (Vrikshasana)

- Begin in Mountain Pose (Fig. 7).
- Let your eyes gaze on a point in front of you and allow your breath to become steady.
- Turn the right knee out and bring the right knee up and set the foot on the left leg
- Level your hips and lift at the heart center.
- Take the arms out to the side and express your tree any way you would like!
- Hold and breathe.
- Repeat other side.

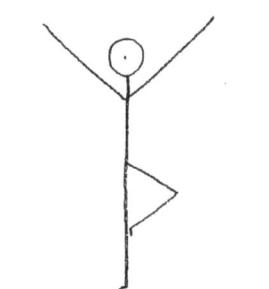

Fig. 44: Tree (Vrikshasana)

Butterfly/Cobbler (Baddha Konasana)

- Come to a comfortable easy-seated pose (Fig. 1).
- Assure yourself that the pelvis and the spine are aligned so that you are sitting comfortably.
- You may wish to set your hands behind you and push firmly into the floor to help steady this position.
- Bring the soles of the feet together.
- On an out-breath, open the inner thighs outward and as the knees move down toward the floor.
- Inhale, let them rise and bring them up.
- Repeat like a butterfly might open and close its wings.
- Hold the outward motion and breathe.

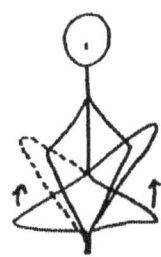

Fig. 45: Butterfly/Cobbler (Baddha Konasana)

Seated Twist (Ardha Matsyendrasana)

- Come to an easy-seated pose with support. (Fig 1).
- Extend the left leg out and bring the right foot to set firmly on the floor next to the left thigh.
- Embrace the right knee with the left hand and take your right hand to press firmly on the floor behind the left hip.
- Adjust the hips so that they are level.
- Feel the heart center lift and the shoulders roll down and back.
- Take a breath and, as you exhale, shift the right hip back and the left hip forward.
- Continue to spiral to the right up the spine, letting your head be the last thing to come around.
- Hold the pose with the arms, shoulders relaxed and the breath filling the right lung completely.
- Rest and breathe.
- Repeat other side.

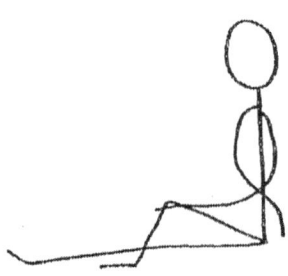

Fig. 46: Seated Twist (Ardha Matsyendrasana)

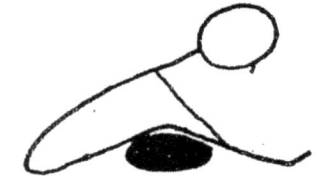

Fig. 47: Seated Supported Forward Fold
(Paschimottanasana)

Seated Supported Forward Fold
(Paschimottanasana)
- Sit on a blanket so the head, neck and trunk are in alignment.
- Place a support under or over your knees until you can fold forward from the hip joint and rest the torso forward.
- Hold and breathe.

The following pages are for you to use to "journal" your daily practice. This may help you become more intentional about your practice. Feel free to copy.

_____ 's Yoga Journal

1. Date: Time: Duration of practice:

2. What are my goals in my physical, emotional, and spiritual practice?

3. Practice Plan
    I'll remember: To practice in the present moment....judging not the past or the future.
                     To practice on the physical, emotional, and spiritual dimension.

    I.   Centering & Warm-up Poses

    II.   Poses for the day
            1.   Heating poses (select standing and back-bending poses)

            2.   Cooling poses (from forward-bending or twisting poses)

    III.   Pranayama/Relaxation/Meditation

    What were my feelings/insights during practice?

    What were my "excuses" for not practicing the way I wanted to?

    What do I need to know more about?

_____ 's Yoga Journal

1. Date: Time: Duration of practice:

2. What are my goals in my physical, emotional, and spiritual practice?

3. Practice Plan
     I'll remember: To practice in the present moment....judging not the past or the future.
                      To practice on the physical, emotional, and spiritual dimension.

   I.   Centering & Warm-up Poses

   II.   Poses for the day
            1.   Heating poses (select standing and back-bending poses)

            2.   Cooling poses (from forward-bending or twisting poses)

   III.   Pranayama/Relaxation/Meditation

What were my feelings/insights during practice?

What were my "excuses" for not practicing the way I wanted to?

What do I need to know more about?

_____'s Yoga Journal

1. Date: Time: Duration of practice:

2. What are my goals in my physical, emotional, and spiritual practice?

3. Practice Plan
   I'll remember: To practice in the present moment....judging not the past or the future.
                     To practice on the physical, emotional, and spiritual dimension.

   I.   Centering & Warm-up Poses

   II.   Poses for the day
           1.   Heating poses (select standing and back-bending poses)

           2.   Cooling poses (from forward-bending or twisting poses)

   III.   Pranayama/Relaxation/Meditation

   What were my feelings/insights during practice?

   What were my "excuses" for not practicing the way I wanted to?

   What do I need to know more about?

_____'s Yoga Journal

1. Date: Time: Duration of practice:

2. What are my goals in my physical, emotional, and spiritual practice?

3. Practice Plan

    I'll remember: To practice in the present moment....judging not the past or the future.

                      To practice on the physical, emotional, and spiritual dimension.

    I.   Centering & Warm-up Poses

    II.   Poses for the day
          1.   Heating poses (select standing and back-bending poses)

          2.   Cooling poses (from forward-bending or twisting poses)

    III.   Pranayama/Relaxation/Meditation

What were my feelings/insights during practice?

What were my "excuses" for not practicing the way I wanted to?

What do I need to know more about?

_____ 's Yoga Journal

1. Date: Time: Duration of practice:

2. What are my goals in my physical, emotional, and spiritual practice?

3. Practice Plan
   I'll remember: To practice in the present moment....judging not the past or the future.
                    To practice on the physical, emotional, and spiritual dimension.

   I.   Centering & Warm-up Poses

   II.   Poses for the day
           1.   Heating poses (select standing and back-bending poses)

           2.   Cooling poses (from forward-bending or twisting poses)

   III.   Pranayama/Relaxation/Meditation

   What were my feelings/insights during practice?

   What were my "excuses" for not practicing the way I wanted to?

   What do I need to know more about?

_____ 's Yoga Journal

1. Date: Time: Duration of practice:

2. What are my goals in my physical, emotional, and spiritual practice?

3. Practice Plan
    I'll remember: To practice in the present moment....judging not the past or the future.
                      To practice on the physical, emotional, and spiritual dimension.

    I.   Centering & Warm-up Poses

    II.   Poses for the day
        1.   Heating poses (select standing and back-bending poses)

        2.   Cooling poses (from forward-bending or twisting poses)

    III.   Pranayama/Relaxation/Meditation

    What were my feelings/insights during practice?

    What were my "excuses" for not practicing the way I wanted to?

    What do I need to know more about?

Trailhead Healing Arts Center is dedicated to creating a dynamic space of community, education, and healing. Trailhead healing arts professionals serve our community with integrity, compassion, and professionalism. Experience and learn about complimentary medicine, meditation, yoga for all levels, yoga teacher training, dance for fitness and emotional health, bodywork, aromatherapy, Reiki, herbal therapy, Ayurvedic medicine, and counseling with our workshops, seminars and holistic clinic.

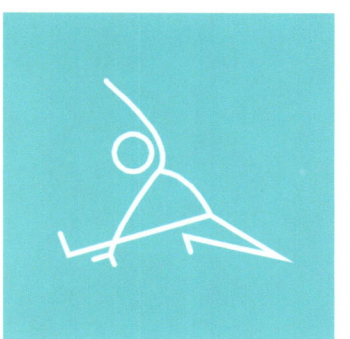

Why the name Trailhead?

So many people have asked us about the name "Trailhead" commenting...." it sounds like an outdoor equipment store."

The trailhead is the place where you get direction, get support, and start your journey. It is a place where you can return to again and again if you get lost or discouraged. This is what we are about...providing you with the tools and support for your journey. We offer the perfect place to support your physical, emotional, and spiritual wellness.

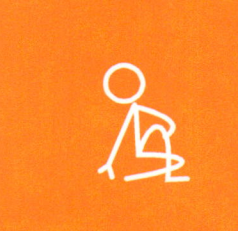

Healing Arts Center

Come and see our beautiful, serene space where a wide variety of healing arts therapies and services are offered to support your wellness and growth.

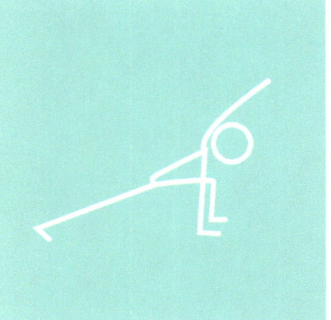

Studio Store

Our store offers fair trade gifts and household items, a selection of natural food items, holistic treasures from around the world, yoga attire, supplies for your yoga/ meditation practice, herbal remedies, books and jewelry.

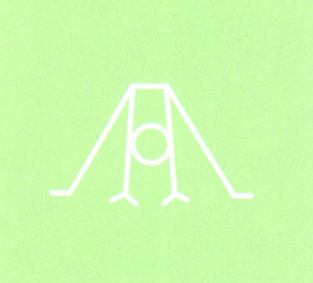

Space for Rent

Trailhead Healing Arts Center rents space to professionals who would like to offer their services to the community.